Intermittent Fasting Unlocked

Your Comprehensive Guide to Achieving Optimal Health and Wellness

Anais Dubreuil

Table of Contents:

Introduction

In today's fast-paced world, where information and lifestyles change rapidly, the pursuit of optimal health and wellness has become a universal aspiration. Amidst this quest, intermittent fasting has emerged as a compelling and transformative approach. Welcome to "Intermittent Fasting Unlocked: Your Comprehensive Guide to Achieving Optimal Health and Wellness."

Intermittent fasting is not just another dietary trend; it is a lifestyle that has captured the attention of health-conscious individuals around the globe. At its core, intermittent fasting is about when you eat, rather than what you eat. By strategically timing your meals and periods of fasting, you can unlock a myriad of health benefits, from weight loss and improved metabolic health to enhanced cognitive function and longevity.

In this comprehensive guide, we will embark on a journey into the world of intermittent fasting, demystifying its science, exploring its diverse approaches, and providing you with the knowledge and tools to incorporate it seamlessly into your life. Whether you're a seasoned fasting enthusiast or a curious newcomer, this book is designed to be your trusted companion, helping you tailor intermittent fasting to your unique needs and goals.

Our 12 chapters will walk you through the fundamentals of intermittent fasting, ranging from understanding the science behind it to customizing your fasting schedule, optimizing your nutrition during eating windows, and even combining intermittent fasting with other dietary approaches. Along the way, we'll address common challenges, provide practical tips, and offer insights to help you sustain your fasting practice in the long run.

As you turn the pages of this book, you'll discover the power of intermittent fasting as a holistic approach to wellness, one that encompasses not only physical health but also mental clarity and emotional balance. We'll equip you with the knowledge and confidence to make informed choices, allowing you to embark on a journey towards a healthier, more vibrant you.

So, whether you're seeking weight loss, improved energy levels, or a path to greater well-being, "Intermittent Fasting Unlocked" is your roadmap to achieving your health and wellness aspirations. Let's begin this transformative journey together, and unlock the incredible potential of intermittent fasting.

Chapter 1: Understanding Intermittent Fasting

Intermittent fasting, often abbreviated as IF, is the cornerstone of a growing movement that has redefined how we approach nutrition and health. In this chapter, we will delve deep into the essence of intermittent fasting, exploring its core principles, the science that underpins it, and the remarkable health benefits it offers.

What Is Intermittent Fasting?

At its essence, intermittent fasting is not a diet in the traditional sense but a pattern of eating. It's a lifestyle approach that involves alternating periods of fasting, where you abstain from calorie intake, with periods of eating. Unlike many diets that focus on what you eat, intermittent fasting primarily concerns itself with when you eat.

Intermittent fasting is flexible, allowing you to choose from various fasting and eating patterns to suit your preferences and goals. Whether you're fasting for 16 hours a day, consuming all your meals within an 8-hour window, or opting for a more extended fast a couple of times a week, the core principle remains the same: cycling between periods of fasting and eating.

The Science Behind It

To understand the power of intermittent fasting, it's crucial to grasp the science that drives it. Fasting triggers a cascade of physiological changes in your body that promote better health. When you abstain from food for an extended period, your body shifts from using glucose as its primary energy source to burning stored fat. This metabolic switch has numerous advantages, including weight loss, improved insulin sensitivity, and reduced inflammation.

Intermittent fasting also stimulates autophagy, a process in which your cells remove damaged components and recycle them, promoting cellular health and longevity. Additionally, fasting can enhance brain function by boosting the production of brain-derived neurotrophic factor (BDNF), a protein that supports cognitive function and mood regulation.

Health Benefits of Intermittent Fasting

The benefits of intermittent fasting extend far beyond weight management. This chapter will introduce you to a range of health advantages that include:

- **Weight Loss:** Intermittent fasting helps you shed excess pounds by creating a calorie deficit and improving fat metabolism.

- **Improved Insulin Sensitivity:** Fasting enhances your body's ability to regulate blood sugar levels, reducing the risk of type 2 diabetes.
- **Heart Health:** Intermittent fasting can lead to lower blood pressure, reduced cholesterol levels, and a decreased risk of heart disease.
- **Enhanced Cognitive Function:** By promoting the growth of new neurons and improving brain health, intermittent fasting can boost your memory, focus, and mental clarity.
- **Longevity:** Emerging research suggests that intermittent fasting may increase lifespan by promoting cellular repair and reducing the risk of age-related diseases.

As we journey through this book, you'll gain a deeper understanding of these benefits and learn how to harness the power of intermittent fasting to achieve your specific health and wellness goals. Prepare to explore the various approaches to intermittent fasting and find the one that best aligns with your lifestyle and aspirations.

Chapter 2: Different Approaches to Fasting

Intermittent fasting offers a world of flexibility when it comes to choosing the fasting pattern that suits your lifestyle and goals. In this chapter, we will explore a range of different approaches to fasting, each with its unique characteristics and potential benefits.

The 16/8 Method

The 16/8 method, also known as the Leangains protocol, is one of the most popular fasting approaches. It involves fasting for 16 hours each day and restricting your eating to an 8-hour window. For example, you might fast from 8 PM to 12 PM the following day and eat your meals between 12 PM and 8 PM. This approach is relatively easy to integrate into your daily routine.

The 5:2 Diet

The 5:2 diet is another well-known fasting strategy. With this approach, you eat regularly for five days a week and significantly reduce your calorie intake (usually around 500-600 calories) on the other two non-consecutive days. While this method may feel more challenging on fasting days, it allows for greater flexibility on regular eating days.

Eat-Stop-Eat

Eat-Stop-Eat involves full-day fasts, typically lasting for 24 hours. You might choose to fast from dinner one day to dinner the next day, creating a 24-hour fasting window. This method is usually practiced 1-2 times a week, providing extended periods of calorie restriction.

Alternate-Day Fasting

As the name suggests, alternate-day fasting involves alternating between fasting days and regular eating days. On fasting days, you either consume very few calories or none at all. This approach can be effective for weight loss but may be challenging for some due to the frequent fasting days.

Warrior Diet

The Warrior Diet is an eating pattern that combines a 20-hour fasting period with a 4-hour eating window in the evening. During the fasting period, small amounts of raw fruits and vegetables or light snacks are allowed. This approach mimics the eating patterns of ancient warriors and emphasizes large, satisfying meals in the evening.

OMAD (One Meal a Day)

OMAD is perhaps one of the most extreme forms of intermittent fasting. As the name suggests, you consume all your daily calories in a single meal, typically within a 1-2 hour window. This method can be challenging but offers an extended fasting period each day.

Throughout this chapter, we will delve deeper into the specifics of each fasting method, discussing their potential benefits, challenges, and who might find each approach most suitable. By understanding these variations, you can tailor your fasting regimen to align with your preferences and achieve your health and wellness objectives.

Chapter 3: Customizing Your Fasting Schedule

Intermittent fasting is not a one-size-fits-all approach; it's a customizable strategy that can be adapted to your unique lifestyle and goals. In this chapter, we'll explore how to personalize your fasting schedule to make intermittent fasting work for you.

Finding the Right Fasting Window

Choosing the fasting window that suits you is a crucial aspect of intermittent fasting. We'll delve into various fasting windows, such as the 16/8 method, 5:2 diet, and others, to help you understand their dynamics and identify the one that aligns best with your daily routine and preferences. Whether you're an early riser or a night owl, there's a fasting window that can fit your lifestyle.

Adapting to Your Lifestyle

Intermittent fasting doesn't mean you have to overhaul your life. We'll discuss strategies for seamlessly integrating fasting into your daily routine, whether you have a busy work schedule, family commitments, or a social life. You'll learn how to navigate social events and outings while maintaining your fasting regimen.

Fasting for Weight Loss

If weight loss is your primary goal, we'll explore fasting strategies that are particularly effective for shedding pounds. You'll discover how intermittent fasting creates a calorie deficit, accelerates fat loss, and helps you achieve your desired weight while preserving muscle mass.

Fasting for Muscle Gain

For those interested in building or maintaining muscle while fasting, we'll provide insights into how to structure your fasting schedule and nutrition to support your fitness goals. Learn the best times to eat to optimize muscle recovery and growth.

Fasting for Mental Clarity

Intermittent fasting isn't just about physical health—it can also sharpen your mental acuity. We'll uncover the science behind how fasting can improve cognitive function, boost focus, and enhance overall brain health. You'll discover how to harness these benefits to excel in your daily tasks.

By the end of this chapter, you'll have the knowledge and tools to craft a fasting schedule that aligns with your lifestyle and objectives. Whether you're fasting for weight management, muscle gain, mental clarity, or a combination of these, understanding how to customize your fasting approach is key to achieving your desired results.

Chapter 4: Getting Started

Now that you have a solid understanding of intermittent fasting and how to customize your fasting schedule, it's time to take the plunge and get started. In this chapter, we will explore the practical steps and considerations for launching your intermittent fasting journey.

Preparing for Your First Fast

Embarking on your first fasting experience can be both exciting and slightly daunting. We'll guide you through the preparations, including setting a start date, clearing your kitchen of temptations, and mentally preparing yourself for the fasting ahead. You'll learn how to set realistic expectations for your initial fasts.

Overcoming Common Challenges

Fasting may present some initial challenges, such as hunger pangs and cravings. We'll provide strategies to overcome these hurdles, including staying hydrated, consuming beverages that support fasting, and using distraction techniques. You'll discover that with the right mindset and tools, you can navigate these challenges successfully.

Staying Hydrated and Nourished

During fasting periods, it's essential to stay properly hydrated and ensure you get the necessary nutrients when you do eat. We'll discuss the importance of water intake, herbal teas, and black coffee while fasting. Additionally, you'll learn how to create balanced meals that provide the nutrients your body needs during eating windows.

Monitoring Your Progress

Tracking your progress is a vital aspect of your fasting journey. We'll explore methods to monitor your weight, body composition, and other relevant metrics. By keeping a journal or using digital tools, you can gain valuable insights into how intermittent fasting is benefiting your health.

As you dive into your fasting journey, remember that it's a process of adaptation. Initial challenges will likely give way to a sense of empowerment and improved well-being. This chapter will equip you with the knowledge and practical tips you need to confidently embark on your intermittent fasting adventure. Whether you're fasting for better health, weight loss, or other personal goals, you're now ready to take the first steps toward a more vibrant and balanced life.

Chapter 5: Nutrition During Eating Windows

While intermittent fasting primarily focuses on when you eat, what you consume during your eating windows plays a pivotal role in maximizing its benefits. In this chapter, we'll delve into the principles of nutrition during your eating periods to support your health and wellness goals.

Building Balanced Meals

Balanced meals are key to ensuring that you get the nutrients your body needs. We'll explore the components of a well-rounded meal, including lean proteins, healthy fats, complex carbohydrates, and plenty of fruits and vegetables. You'll discover how to create satisfying and nourishing meals that promote overall well-being.

Nutrient-Rich Foods

Certain foods provide a more significant nutritional punch than others. We'll identify nutrient-dense foods that can help you meet your dietary needs while keeping your calorie intake in check. You'll learn to make the most of your eating windows by incorporating these foods into your meals.

Avoiding Overindulgence

Intermittent fasting can provide a sense of freedom during eating windows, but it's crucial to avoid overindulgence. We'll discuss mindful eating techniques, portion control, and strategies to prevent excessive calorie intake. You'll gain insights into how to strike a balance between enjoying your meals and maintaining your health goals.

Meal Timing and Composition

The timing and composition of your meals can impact your fasting experience. We'll explore the benefits of specific meal timing strategies, such as consuming higher-carb or higher-protein meals. You'll learn how to optimize your eating patterns to align with your goals, whether they involve weight loss, muscle gain, or enhanced cognitive function.

Hydration and Supplements

Proper hydration is essential during eating windows, and we'll discuss the role of water, herbal teas, and other beverages in supporting your nutritional needs. Additionally, we'll touch on dietary supplements that may complement your fasting regimen, including vitamins, minerals, and other micronutrients.

By the end of this chapter, you'll have a comprehensive understanding of how to make the most of your eating windows during intermittent fasting. You'll be equipped with the knowledge to create satisfying, nutrient-dense meals and use meal timing to your advantage. With these insights, you can ensure that your nutritional choices align with your health and wellness goals while practicing intermittent fasting.

Chapter 6: Fasting and Exercise

Integrating exercise with intermittent fasting can amplify the benefits of both practices. In this chapter, we will explore how to effectively combine fasting with various forms of physical activity to optimize your health and fitness goals.

Exercising While Fasting

Fasting and exercise can go hand in hand, but it's essential to understand the nuances of working out in a fasted state. We'll delve into the advantages of fasting for exercise, such as enhanced fat burning and improved insulin sensitivity. You'll learn how to structure your workouts during fasting periods to maximize these benefits.

Maximizing Fat Burn

Fasting can boost your body's ability to burn fat, making it an excellent companion for those aiming to shed pounds. We'll discuss the science behind fasting-induced fat loss and provide exercise strategies that harness this effect. You'll discover how to leverage fasting to accelerate your weight loss journey.

Workout Timing Strategies

Timing your workouts strategically can make a significant difference in your fasting experience. We'll explore different workout timing options, including exercising before or after eating, and their impact on your energy levels and performance. You'll gain insights into tailoring your exercise routine to align with your fasting schedule.

Nutrition for Active Fasters

Maintaining proper nutrition is crucial when you're both fasting and exercising. We'll discuss the nutrients your body needs to fuel workouts and recover effectively. You'll learn how to plan your meals to support your exercise routine and overall health.

Hydration and Recovery

Staying hydrated is vital during exercise, especially when fasting. We'll provide guidance on how to ensure you're adequately hydrated while respecting your fasting windows. Additionally, we'll cover post-workout recovery strategies, including the timing of meals and the importance of protein intake.

By the end of this chapter, you'll have a comprehensive understanding of how to integrate exercise seamlessly into your intermittent fasting routine. Whether you're aiming to boost fat burn, improve muscle tone, or enhance your overall fitness, you'll be well-equipped to leverage the synergy between fasting and exercise to reach your goals.

Chapter 7: Monitoring Progress

As you continue your intermittent fasting practice, it's essential to monitor your progress to ensure you're on the right track and making the most of this lifestyle. In this chapter, we'll explore various methods and tools for tracking your fasting journey and making informed adjustments.

Tracking Your Results

Measuring your results is a fundamental aspect of intermittent fasting. We'll discuss key metrics to monitor, such as weight, body composition, and waist circumference. You'll learn how to use these metrics to assess your progress over time and set realistic goals.

Keeping a Fasting Journal

Maintaining a fasting journal can provide valuable insights into your habits, challenges, and successes. We'll guide you on how to keep a comprehensive fasting journal, including recording your fasting and eating windows, daily energy levels, mood, and any notable observations. This practice can help you identify patterns and make data-driven decisions.

Digital Tools and Apps

In the digital age, there is an abundance of apps and tools designed to assist with intermittent fasting. We'll explore popular fasting apps that can help you track your fasting windows, set reminders, and log your meals. These tools can simplify the tracking process and provide a visual representation of your fasting journey.

Making Adjustments as Needed

Intermittent fasting is not static; it can and should evolve as your goals and circumstances change. We'll discuss the importance of being adaptable and making adjustments when necessary. Whether you need to tweak your fasting schedule, modify your meal composition, or alter your exercise routine, you'll gain the knowledge to fine-tune your fasting regimen.

Recognizing Plateaus

Plateaus are a common occurrence in any wellness journey, including intermittent fasting. We'll explore why plateaus happen and how to overcome them. By understanding the potential roadblocks and implementing strategies to break through them, you can continue progressing towards your goals.

By the end of this chapter, you'll be well-versed in tracking your intermittent fasting progress and equipped with the tools to ensure you stay motivated and on course. Monitoring your journey not only helps you celebrate your successes but also empowers you to make informed decisions that align with your health and wellness objectives.

Chapter 8: Combining Fasting with Other Diets

Intermittent fasting can be seamlessly integrated with various dietary approaches to create a synergy that enhances your overall health and wellness. In this chapter, we will explore how to combine intermittent fasting with different diets to meet specific goals and preferences.

Keto and Intermittent Fasting

The ketogenic (keto) diet and intermittent fasting share common ground in promoting fat metabolism and weight loss. We'll discuss how these two strategies complement each other, providing insights into achieving and maintaining a state of ketosis while fasting. Learn how to harness the synergy of keto and intermittent fasting for enhanced fat loss and improved metabolic health.

Vegan and Intermittent Fasting

Veganism and intermittent fasting may seem like an unlikely pair, but they can coexist harmoniously. We'll explore plant-based fasting options and offer guidance on ensuring you meet your nutritional needs during eating windows. Discover how to reap the benefits of both approaches while adhering to your ethical and dietary choices.

Paleo and Intermittent Fasting

The paleo diet, which focuses on whole, unprocessed foods, can align beautifully with intermittent fasting. We'll explore how these two dietary philosophies complement each other and provide guidelines for combining them effectively. Learn how to create paleo-friendly meals within your fasting and eating windows.

Mediterranean Diet and Intermittent Fasting

The Mediterranean diet, renowned for its heart-healthy benefits, can be enhanced by intermittent fasting. We'll discuss how to incorporate Mediterranean-style meals into your fasting and eating windows. Discover the potential synergy between these two approaches in promoting cardiovascular health and overall well-being.

By the end of this chapter, you'll have a comprehensive understanding of how to combine intermittent fasting with various dietary styles to achieve your specific health and wellness objectives. Whether you're looking to boost weight loss, improve metabolic health, or align your fasting practice with your dietary preferences, you'll be well-prepared to

create a balanced and customized approach that suits
your needs.

Chapter 9: Fasting for Specific Goals

Intermittent fasting can be tailored to address specific health and wellness goals, providing a versatile tool for personal growth and improvement. In this chapter, we will explore how to harness the power of intermittent fasting to achieve targeted objectives.

Fasting for Longevity

Extending lifespan and promoting healthy aging are aspirations shared by many. We'll delve into the science of fasting for longevity, including the mechanisms by which intermittent fasting may support cellular repair and reduce the risk of age-related diseases. Discover strategies for incorporating fasting into your life to maximize its potential longevity benefits.

Fasting for Diabetes Management

Intermittent fasting has shown promise in helping individuals manage and prevent type 2 diabetes. We'll explore how fasting can improve insulin sensitivity, regulate blood sugar levels, and reduce the risk of diabetic complications. Learn how to implement fasting as a complementary strategy in your diabetes management plan.

Fasting for Heart Health

Heart health is of paramount importance, and intermittent fasting can play a role in maintaining cardiovascular wellness. We'll discuss the impact of fasting on blood pressure, cholesterol levels, and other heart-related factors. Discover how to tailor your fasting regimen to support a heart-healthy lifestyle.

Fasting for Cognitive Function

A sharp and agile mind is essential for a fulfilling life. Intermittent fasting has been linked to improved cognitive function and brain health. We'll explore the science behind fasting's effects on the brain and provide insights into how to optimize your fasting practice to boost mental clarity, focus, and memory.

By the end of this chapter, you'll have a deep understanding of how to use intermittent fasting as a targeted approach to address specific health and wellness goals. Whether you're focused on extending your lifespan, managing a medical condition, or enhancing cognitive function, you'll be empowered to leverage intermittent fasting as a valuable tool on your journey to well-being.

Chapter 10: Overcoming Challenges and Side Effects

Embarking on an intermittent fasting journey may not always be smooth sailing. In this chapter, we will explore common challenges and potential side effects that may arise during your fasting practice. More importantly, we'll provide strategies to overcome these hurdles effectively.

Dealing with Hunger and Cravings

Hunger pangs and food cravings are among the most prevalent challenges encountered during fasting. We'll delve into the physiological and psychological aspects of hunger, offering practical techniques to manage and minimize these sensations. Discover how to build resilience and maintain self-control when faced with cravings.

Managing Digestive Issues

Some individuals may experience digestive discomfort while fasting. We'll explore potential digestive issues such as acid reflux, constipation, or indigestion, and provide strategies to alleviate these concerns. Learn how to promote digestive health while practicing intermittent fasting.

Avoiding Nutritional Deficiencies

Ensuring you meet your nutritional needs is crucial for long-term well-being. We'll discuss how to maintain a balanced diet that provides essential vitamins, minerals, and other nutrients during your eating windows. You'll gain insights into potential deficiencies that may arise and how to address them.

Handling Social Situations

Navigating social events, family gatherings, and outings with friends can pose challenges for intermittent fasters. We'll offer practical tips for maintaining your fasting regimen while enjoying a vibrant social life. Discover strategies for communicating your fasting choices to others and managing peer pressure effectively.

By the end of this chapter, you'll be equipped with a toolbox of strategies to overcome challenges and navigate potential side effects that may arise during your intermittent fasting journey. With the right knowledge and mindset, you can confidently address these obstacles, ensuring a smooth and successful fasting practice.

Chapter 11: Sustainability and Lifestyle

The long-term success of intermittent fasting hinges on its sustainability within the context of your unique lifestyle. In this chapter, we will explore strategies for integrating intermittent fasting seamlessly into your daily routine, making it a sustainable and enduring part of your lifestyle.

Making Intermittent Fasting a Habit

Sustainability begins with forming lasting habits. We'll delve into the psychology of habit formation and provide practical tips for embedding intermittent fasting into your daily life. Discover how to build a strong foundation for a sustainable fasting practice.

Fasting While Traveling

Travel can present unique challenges for intermittent fasters. We'll offer guidance on maintaining your fasting routine when you're on the go, whether for work or leisure. Learn how to adapt your fasting schedule to different time zones and navigate travel-related food choices.

Fasting and Social Life

Balancing intermittent fasting with social engagements is key to long-term sustainability. We'll explore strategies for enjoying social events, dining out, and celebrating special occasions while adhering to your fasting goals. Discover how to harmonize your social life with your fasting lifestyle.

Embracing Flexibility

Sustainability doesn't mean rigidity. We'll discuss the importance of flexibility within your fasting practice. You'll learn how to adapt your fasting schedule when life throws unexpected challenges your way, ensuring that your fasting journey remains adaptable and sustainable.

Maintaining a Healthy Relationship with Food

Intuitive eating and a positive relationship with food are integral to sustainability. We'll delve into the concept of mindful eating and offer guidance on listening to your body's hunger and satiety cues. Discover how to foster a balanced approach to food that aligns with your fasting goals.

By the end of this chapter, you'll be well-prepared to make intermittent fasting a sustainable and harmonious part of your lifestyle. Sustainability is the key to reaping the long-term benefits of intermittent fasting while enjoying the flexibility to adapt to life's ever-changing demands and opportunities.

Chapter 12: Celebrating Your Success

As you near the end of this journey, it's essential to recognize and celebrate your fasting accomplishments. In this chapter, we'll explore the art of self-reflection and goal setting, helping you acknowledge how far you've come and plan for your fasting future.

Reflecting on Your Journey

Self-reflection is a powerful tool for personal growth. We'll guide you in looking back on your intermittent fasting journey, encouraging you to celebrate the milestones you've achieved and the challenges you've overcome. Embrace the opportunity to learn from your experiences and apply those lessons moving forward.

Setting New Goals

Fasting is a dynamic practice that can evolve with your changing aspirations. We'll discuss how to set new, meaningful goals for your fasting practice, whether they involve further weight loss, improved fitness, enhanced mental clarity, or other objectives. Discover how to define clear and achievable goals to keep you motivated.

Maintaining a Healthy Relationship with Food

Your relationship with food plays a central role in your fasting success. We'll revisit the importance of maintaining a balanced and positive connection with food. Learn how to continue practicing mindful eating and making food choices that align with your long-term well-being.

Continuing Your Fasting Journey

Your fasting journey doesn't have to end here. We'll provide guidance on how to continue fasting as an enduring part of your lifestyle. Explore strategies for refining your fasting schedule, incorporating variety, and sustaining your newfound habits.

Sharing Your Success

Sharing your success with others can be incredibly motivating and inspiring. We'll discuss how to communicate your fasting achievements with friends and family, and perhaps even encourage them to embark on their own fasting journeys. Your success can ripple out to benefit those around you.

By the end of this chapter, you'll be ready to embrace and celebrate your intermittent fasting accomplishments, armed with the tools to continue your journey in a sustainable and fulfilling manner. Remember that intermittent fasting is not just a practice; it's a lifestyle that can positively influence your overall health and well-being for years to come.

Conclusion

As you reach the end of "Intermittent Fasting Unlocked: Your Comprehensive Guide to Achieving Optimal Health and Wellness," you've embarked on a transformative journey into the world of intermittent fasting. You've explored the science, various fasting approaches, and practical strategies to make this powerful lifestyle work for you.

Intermittent fasting isn't just about when you eat; it's a holistic approach to wellness that encompasses physical health, mental clarity, and emotional balance. By incorporating intermittent fasting into your life, you've taken a significant step toward achieving your health and wellness aspirations.

Remember that your intermittent fasting journey is uniquely yours. Whether you're fasting for weight loss, improved metabolic health, muscle gain, enhanced cognitive function, or other specific goals, the knowledge and tools you've gained in this guide can be customized to meet your needs.

As you move forward, embrace the power of self-reflection, goal setting, and maintaining a healthy relationship with food. Continue to celebrate your achievements, both big and small, and share your success with others to inspire and motivate those around you.

Your journey doesn't end here; it's an ongoing exploration of well-being and vitality. As you continue your intermittent fasting practice, may you find fulfillment, balance, and a renewed sense of health and vitality. With the knowledge and tools you've acquired, you're well-equipped to unlock the incredible potential of intermittent fasting and enjoy a life of optimal health and wellness.

Thank you for joining us on this journey, and may your path be filled with health, happiness, and the fulfillment of your goals.

Appendix: Meal Plans

In this appendix, you will find practical meal plans tailored to various intermittent fasting styles and goals. These meal plans provide clear examples of what to eat during fasting and eating windows. Please note that these plans are flexible and can be adjusted based on your preferences and dietary requirements.

Meal Plan 1: 16/8 Intermittent Fasting

- **Fasting Window (16 hours):** 8:00 PM - 12:00 PM
- **Eating Window (8 hours):** 12:00 PM - 8:00 PM

Sample Meals:

- **Lunch (12:00 PM):** Grilled chicken breast with mixed greens salad (olive oil and balsamic vinegar dressing).
- **Snack (3:00 PM):** Greek yogurt with berries and almonds.
- **Dinner (6:30 PM):** Baked salmon with steamed broccoli and quinoa.
- **Optional Snack (7:30 PM):** Sliced cucumber with hummus.

Meal Plan 2: 5:2 Intermittent Fasting (Fasting Day)

- **Fasting Window (24 hours):** Full Day

Sample Meals:

- **Breakfast:** Herbal tea or black coffee (no sugar or cream).
- **Lunch:** Vegetable broth-based soup with a side salad (light on dressing).
- **Snack:** A small handful of almonds or walnuts.
- **Dinner:** Grilled or roasted vegetables with a portion of lean protein (e.g., grilled chicken or tofu).
- **Evening:** Herbal tea or water.

Meal Plan 3: OMAD (One Meal a Day) Intermittent Fasting

- **Fasting Window (23 hours):** 1 hour

Sample Meal:

- **6:00 PM:** A well-balanced meal with lean protein, plenty of vegetables, and healthy fats (e.g., grilled salmon, asparagus, and avocado).

Meal Plan 4: Intermittent Fasting and Exercise

- **Fasting Window (16 hours):** 8:00 PM - 12:00 PM

- **Eating Window (8 hours):** 12:00 PM - 8:00 PM

Sample Meals:

- **Pre-workout Snack (10:00 AM):** Banana and a handful of almonds.
- **Post-workout Meal (12:00 PM):** Protein-rich lunch (e.g., turkey and avocado wrap with whole-grain bread).
- **Snack (3:00 PM):** Greek yogurt with honey.
- **Dinner (6:30 PM):** Grilled lean steak with sweet potato and steamed broccoli.

Meal Plan 5: Balanced Intermittent Fasting Meal

- **Fasting Window (14 hours):** 10:00 PM - 12:00 PM
- **Eating Window (10 hours):** 12:00 PM - 10:00 PM

Sample Meals:

- **Breakfast (8:00 AM):** Scrambled eggs with spinach, tomatoes, whole-grain toast, and a small fruit salad.
- **Lunch (12:30 PM):** Grilled chicken breast with quinoa, mixed vegetables, and a light vinaigrette.

- **Snack (3:30 PM):** Greek yogurt with sliced strawberries.
- **Dinner (7:00 PM):** Baked salmon with brown rice and steamed asparagus.

These meal plans are practical examples to help structure your meals during intermittent fasting. Adjust portion sizes and food choices based on your needs and preferences. Consult a healthcare professional or registered dietitian for personalized guidance, especially if you have specific dietary concerns or health conditions.

Appendix: Recipes

In this appendix, you'll find a collection of delicious and nutritious recipes designed to support your intermittent fasting journey. These recipes are tailored to various fasting methods and can help you create satisfying meals during your eating windows. Feel free to explore and enjoy these culinary delights as you embark on your intermittent fasting adventure. Remember that these recipes can be adjusted to suit your personal preferences and dietary needs.

1. Protein-Packed Breakfast Bowl

Ingredients:

- 1/2 cup of Greek yogurt
- 1/4 cup of rolled oats
- 1 tablespoon of chia seeds
- 1/2 cup of mixed berries
- 1 tablespoon of honey (optional)
- A sprinkle of almonds or walnuts

Instructions:

1. In a bowl, mix Greek yogurt, rolled oats, and chia seeds.

2. Top with mixed berries and drizzle honey if desired.
3. Sprinkle with almonds or walnuts for added crunch.

2. Mediterranean Quinoa Salad

Ingredients:

- 1 cup of cooked quinoa
- 1/2 cup of cherry tomatoes, halved
- 1/2 cucumber, diced
- 1/4 cup of Kalamata olives, pitted and sliced
- 1/4 cup of feta cheese, crumbled
- 2 tablespoons of extra-virgin olive oil
- 1 tablespoon of fresh lemon juice
- Fresh basil leaves for garnish
- Salt and pepper to taste

Instructions:

1. In a large bowl, combine cooked quinoa, cherry tomatoes, cucumber, olives, and feta cheese.
2. In a small bowl, whisk together olive oil, lemon juice, salt, and pepper.
3. Drizzle the dressing over the salad and toss to combine.
4. Garnish with fresh basil leaves before serving.

3. Grilled Chicken with Lemon and Herbs

Ingredients:

- 2 boneless, skinless chicken breasts
- 2 tablespoons of olive oil
- 1 lemon, juiced and zested
- 2 cloves of garlic, minced
- 1 teaspoon of dried oregano
- Salt and pepper to taste
- Fresh parsley for garnish

Instructions:

1. In a bowl, mix olive oil, lemon juice, lemon zest, minced garlic, dried oregano, salt, and pepper.
2. Marinate chicken breasts in the mixture for at least 30 minutes.
3. Preheat grill or grill pan over medium-high heat.
4. Grill chicken for 6-8 minutes on each side until fully cooked.
5. Garnish with fresh parsley before serving.

4. Berry and Spinach Smoothie

Ingredients:

- 1 cup of spinach leaves
- 1/2 cup of mixed berries (strawberries, blueberries, raspberries)
- 1/2 banana
- 1 cup of almond milk (or any preferred milk)

- 1 tablespoon of honey (optional)
- Ice cubes (optional)

Instructions:

1. Place spinach, mixed berries, banana, almond milk, and honey in a blender.
2. Blend until smooth and creamy.
3. Add ice cubes for a chilled smoothie, if desired.

5. Roasted Vegetable Medley

Ingredients:

- Assorted vegetables (e.g., bell peppers, zucchini, carrots, broccoli)
- 2 tablespoons of olive oil
- Salt and pepper to taste
- Fresh herbs (e.g., rosemary, thyme, or basil) for garnish

Instructions:

1. Preheat the oven to 425°F (220°C).
2. Cut assorted vegetables into bite-sized pieces.
3. Toss the vegetables with olive oil, salt, and pepper.
4. Spread them on a baking sheet in a single layer.
5. Roast for 20-25 minutes or until tender and slightly caramelized.

6. Garnish with fresh herbs before serving.

6. Baked Salmon with Dill Sauce

Ingredients:

- 2 salmon fillets
- 1 tablespoon olive oil
- Salt and pepper to taste
- 1 lemon, thinly sliced
- Fresh dill for garnish

For the Dill Sauce:

- 1/2 cup Greek yogurt
- 1 tablespoon fresh dill, chopped
- 1 teaspoon Dijon mustard
- 1 teaspoon lemon juice
- Salt and pepper to taste

Instructions:

1. Preheat the oven to 375°F (190°C).
2. Place salmon fillets on a baking sheet, drizzle with olive oil, and season with salt and pepper.
3. Lay lemon slices on top of the salmon.
4. Bake for 15-20 minutes or until salmon flakes easily with a fork.
5. While the salmon bakes, mix all the dill sauce ingredients in a bowl.

6. Serve the baked salmon with dill sauce and garnish with fresh dill.

7. Veggie-Packed Omelette

Ingredients:

- 3 eggs
- 1/4 cup bell peppers, diced
- 1/4 cup tomatoes, diced
- 1/4 cup spinach, chopped
- 2 tablespoons onion, diced
- Salt and pepper to taste
- 1 tablespoon olive oil

Instructions:

1. In a bowl, whisk the eggs and season with salt and pepper.
2. Heat olive oil in a non-stick skillet over medium heat.
3. Add diced vegetables and sauté until tender.
4. Pour the whisked eggs over the vegetables and cook until the edges are set.
5. Gently fold the omelette in half and cook for another minute.
6. Slide the omelette onto a plate and serve hot.

8. Quinoa and Black Bean Salad

Ingredients:

- 1 cup cooked quinoa
- 1 cup black beans, drained and rinsed
- 1 cup corn kernels (fresh or frozen)
- 1/2 cup cherry tomatoes, halved
- 1/4 cup red onion, finely chopped
- 1/4 cup fresh cilantro, chopped
- Juice of 1 lime
- 2 tablespoons olive oil
- Salt and pepper to taste

Instructions:

1. In a large bowl, combine cooked quinoa, black beans, corn, cherry tomatoes, red onion, and cilantro.
2. In a small bowl, whisk together lime juice, olive oil, salt, and pepper.
3. Drizzle the dressing over the salad and toss to combine.
4. Serve chilled as a refreshing side dish or a light meal.

9. Avocado and Chickpea Salad

Ingredients:

- 1 ripe avocado, diced
- 1 can chickpeas, drained and rinsed
- 1/4 cup red onion, finely chopped
- 1/4 cup cucumber, diced

- 2 tablespoons fresh parsley, chopped
- Juice of 1 lemon
- 2 tablespoons olive oil
- Salt and pepper to taste

Instructions:

1. In a large bowl, combine diced avocado, chickpeas, red onion, cucumber, and fresh parsley.
2. In a small bowl, whisk together lemon juice, olive oil, salt, and pepper.
3. Drizzle the dressing over the salad and gently toss to coat.
4. Enjoy this refreshing and protein-packed salad.

10. Greek-Style Chicken and Vegetable Skewers

Ingredients:

- 2 boneless, skinless chicken breasts, cut into cubes
- 1 bell pepper, cut into chunks
- 1 red onion, cut into chunks
- Cherry tomatoes
- Wooden skewers (pre-soaked in water)
- 2 tablespoons olive oil
- 2 cloves garlic, minced
- 1 teaspoon dried oregano
- Salt and pepper to taste

- Greek yogurt for dipping (optional)

Instructions:

1. In a bowl, mix olive oil, minced garlic, dried oregano, salt, and pepper.
2. Thread chicken cubes, bell pepper, red onion, and cherry tomatoes onto the soaked wooden skewers.
3. Brush the skewers with the olive oil mixture.
4. Grill or broil the skewers for about 10-15 minutes or until the chicken is cooked through and the vegetables are tender.
5. Serve with Greek yogurt for dipping, if desired.

11. Spinach and Feta Stuffed Mushrooms

Ingredients:

- Large mushrooms (portobello or button)
- 1 cup fresh spinach, chopped
- 1/2 cup feta cheese, crumbled
- 2 cloves garlic, minced
- 2 tablespoons olive oil
- Salt and pepper to taste
- Fresh parsley for garnish

Instructions:

1. Preheat the oven to 375°F (190°C).

2. Remove the stems from the mushrooms and brush the caps with olive oil.
3. In a pan, sauté chopped spinach and minced garlic in olive oil until wilted.
4. Stir in crumbled feta cheese.
5. Stuff the mushroom caps with the spinach and feta mixture.
6. Bake for 15-20 minutes or until the mushrooms are tender.
7. Garnish with fresh parsley before serving.

12. Cucumber and Avocado Salad

Ingredients:

- 2 cucumbers, thinly sliced
- 1 avocado, diced
- 1/4 cup red onion, finely chopped
- 2 tablespoons fresh dill, chopped
- Juice of 1 lime
- 2 tablespoons olive oil
- Salt and pepper to taste

Instructions:

1. In a large bowl, combine sliced cucumbers, diced avocado, red onion, and fresh dill.
2. In a small bowl, whisk together lime juice, olive oil, salt, and pepper.

3. Drizzle the dressing over the salad and gently toss to combine.
4. This refreshing salad is ready to serve.

13. Berry and Nut Parfait

Ingredients:

- Greek yogurt
- Mixed berries (strawberries, blueberries, raspberries)
- Mixed nuts (almonds, walnuts, pecans)
- Honey (optional)

Instructions:

1. In a glass or bowl, layer Greek yogurt, mixed berries, and mixed nuts.
2. Drizzle honey on top if desired.
3. Repeat the layers as needed.
4. Enjoy a nutrient-packed parfait as a satisfying snack or dessert.

These recipes are just a starting point for creating delicious meals during your intermittent fasting journey. Feel free to adapt them to your taste and dietary preferences. Enjoy your culinary adventures while maintaining a healthy fasting lifestyle.

www.ingramcontent.com/pod-product-compliance
Lightning Source LLC
Chambersburg PA
CBHW071118260726
48661CB00006B/2645